VITALITY

A Holistic and
Natural
Approach to
Health

By Michael Jones

Table Of Contents
INTRODUCTION

CONCLUSION

ABOUT THE AUTHOR

INTRODUCTION

Have you found it difficult to lose weight, get better sleep, get off of pharmaceutical drugs, or just be healthy overall? If so then you are just like millions of people worldwide that the pharmaceutical industry and the MD's have let down. Over the past century, under the care and guidance of the worlds dominating healthcare organizations, the world's population has become more and more sick. The rates of cancer, autism and obesity, just to name a few, have continually risen every year since the early 1900's, and with so much information available about health, it can become a daunting task to know exactly what is right for you. It is for this reason that I've written this guide to VITALITY . In this book you will learn about the importance of cholesterol. You will learn about the 12 bad foods. You will learn techniques that allow you to heal your body and become the greatest expression of yourself that you could ever dream to be. Inside the pages of "VITALITY" is where you will begin to find your own vitality. So what are you waiting for? Let's get to Chapter 1!

The Dangers of Gluten

In 2018 if you live in the US then you have surely heard of the word gluten and the term "gluten free." Most grocery stores now have gluten free sections and most restaurants offer some sort of gluten free options on their menus. The term "gluten free" has become so popular that it is now mostly just a marketing claim that food companies use to advertise their products. I've even seen gluten free water, which is absolutely ridiculous. In this chapter we will learn exactly what gluten is. What foods contain gluten. Why do these foods contain gluten. The health risks associated with consuming gluten. What the term "gluten free" really means and what are the healthy alternatives to consuming gluten.

Gluten is a protein that is found in wheat, barley, rye and oats. It is a latin word that means glue. Gluten is the "sticky stuff" that gives elasticity to flours, doughs and pasta and holds them together. For this cause, gluten containing grains can be used for a plethora of uses. The use of these grains as food, in particular wheat, can be traced to about 8800 BCE in and around Egypt. By the 15th century wheat and these other grains had spread all the way to the Americas as crops to be used as food. During the industrial revolution the process of making bread sped up tremendously which means wheat was now more accessible to a larger number of people, which also increased its demand. It was this demand that forced scientist to find a faster way to cultivate the grain. This is now the beginning of GMO wheat. Through the process of cross breeding wheat crops to maximize production and ultimately increase profits, the crop has diminished in size to about 2 feet. This has caused the gluten to be concentrated in such a way that this harmless protein is now deadly.

In order to fully understand why this is so bad, we must first have a basic knowledge of proteins, digestion and absorption. I am going to borrow the analogy of Dr Peter Glidden ND to explain this. Let's look at a protein as if it were a pearl necklace. When you consume protein it is the job of the stomach, in particular the stomach acid, to break the bond between each pearl and liberate its molecules. So then you have individual molecules flowing through your digestive tract that eventually end up at your small intestines, where they are absorbed into the body to be used as nutrients. However, in the case of gluten, upwards of 80% of the world's populations stomach acid is not strong enough to break those bonds of the protein molecule. So instead of individual pearls tumbling through your digestive tract, you instead have an entire necklace, or protein, tumbling through and wreaking havoc on your digestive tract and eventually ending up at your small intestines. Your small intestines then tries to absorb this giant molecule , but not only can it not absorb the protein, the molecule destroys your small intestines, which is the beginning of sickness in the body. Linus Pauling, an American Chemist and Biochemist who won the Nobel Prize for Chemistry, once said that all chronic disease could be linked to a mineral deficiency and since gluten, by means of destroying the small intestines, creates deficiencies, then it could be said that gluten plays a very important role in the development of any and all chronic disease. This phenomenon is known as non celiac gluten sensitivity and there is absolutely no MD related test for it.

In her dissertation Pamela Stackhouse MS, HD quoted the work of Ergün, Urhan, and Ayer (2017) as well as the work of Dohan (1966) both studies pointed to the association of celiac disease and schizophrenia. In 2011, cardiologist Dr. William Davis published "Wheat Belly." Dr. Davis is a strong advocate against gluten containing grains. Claiming that avoiding gluten is the way to a happier and healthier life.

Wheat, barley, rye and oats are apart of so many foods that the idea of going gluten free could seem a little bit overwhelming, not to mention understanding how to tell the difference between truly gluten free products and products that are simply advertised as gluten free. However, the transition to gluten free can be very easy and simple to do with just a few tips. Tip number 1. Most restaurants have gluten free options on their menus. Simply take the time to ask if that option is available. Tip number 2. The term "gluten free" appearing within the name of a product is marketing. A quick glance at the label will tell you if the food is really gluten free. Check the ingredients, if you see wheat, barley ,rye or oats, in any form, then the product is not gluten free. Tips number 3. Find a good brand of gluten free products that taste good to you. At the end of this book, I'm going to leave a list of the brands that I use for bread, pasta, cakes and etc.

In closing I want to be sure that you understand that when I speak of gluten that I am speaking solely on wheat, barley,rye and oats that are produced in the US. I do not know enough about wheat production in other countries to speak intelligently on the topic.

The Need For Cholesterol

The need for Cholesterol? Now I understand that this statement goes totally against everything that you have been taught about cholesterol by Medical Doctors but I am going to clear up the misinformation. In understanding the need for cholesterol we must first understand why talking to a Medical Doctor about cholesterol is the equivalent to talking to the wall. The information that they both give will be equally as valuable. The term "Medical Doctor" is a misnomer, it is not real. They simply do not exist. Allow me to explain it this way. If an individual studies Chiropractic then he or she will someday become a Chiropractor. If the same individual, instead studies Naturopathic Medicine then one day that person will become a Naturopath Doctor. In the same way if a person, like myself, studies Holistic Medicine, then they would be considered a

Holistic Health Coach. However, if an individual studies Allopathic Medicine, which is how to treat symptoms with drugs, then they are called a Medical Doctor. MD's do not study or learn about medicine. They learn drugs, how to handle trauma, and some learn surgery. MD's are not required to take any courses on nutrition, herbs or supplements. Yet these are the people that we go to for the symptoms of chronic disease. Your MD may be the nicest person on earth, but when it comes to things like cholesterol and chronic disease, they just do not have a clue, they simply were not trained to.

The first misconception about cholesterol is that it is the same thing as HDL, LDL, or VLDL. HDL stands for high density lipoprotein. LDL stands for low density lipoprotein and VLDL stands for very low density lipoprotein. They are all lipoproteins. Cholesterol is a sterol. Without getting into to much science and complicating things, I think we can just safely determine that based on name alone, lipoproteins and cholesterol are not the same thing. Before I get into the role that these lipoproteins play in the whole cholesterol conversation let me first tell you that your body, by means of your liver, makes cholesterol. So that makes cholesterol a naturally compound within the human body. Here is a quick side note, Statin Drugs, the drugs that MD's prescribe to lower a patient's cholesterol, does so by disrupting the natural production of cholesterol in the liver. This is why if you take a Statin then you have to have your liver checked every six months to check for Hepatitis C.

Now let's take a brief look at the function of the lipoproteins. Cholesterol is dumped into the blood via three different mechanisms. The first is from your liver. Low density lipoproteins (LDL) bring cholesterol from the liver to be used by the cells and tissues of the body. Once that process has ended, it is the job of the high density lipoproteins to collect the cholesterol and return it to the liver so that the process can restart again. Simply stated, the process is like a bus station. The final way that cholesterol enters the bloodstream is by your diet, what you eat. This cholesterol is identical to the cholesterol produced by your liver and follows the same current and process.

Now that we understand what cholesterol is and what it is not, we can now move on to its importance. As I stated earlier, your liver makes cholesterol, but only about 10% of your bodies daily needs. The rest must be consumed and since plant cholesterol, better known as, phytosterol, is toxic to the body in that it interrupts cholesterol, the only sources of dietary cholesterol are from animal sources. I am well aware that my previous statement will be met with opposition from vegetarians and vegans, and one day i'll write an entire ebook on the vegetarian and vegan diets, but for now i'll simply accept that my statement of facts will not be accepted by all. Onto my point. The human brain is makes of about 2% of the body's total weight, but contains about 20% of the body's total cholesterol. The brain is almost 80% pure cholesterol. The human nervous system is entirely made almost entirely of cholesterol. You are made up of somewhere around 70-100 trillion cells, each cell wall is entirely made of cholesterol. To put that plainly, you literally could not exist without cholesterol because you can not have a cell without it. All sex hormones are made of cholesterol and without cholesterol your body cannot make Vitamin D. So basically, when you drive cholesterol into the ground, either by your dietary choices or statin drugs, then you immediately put yourself at risk for Alzheimer's, which is "drying" up of the brain. Low testosterone. Menopause that seems to go on forever and an inability to synthesis Vitamin D. Again, I do realize that there are those that will say that cholesterol causes things like atherosclerosis, or hardening of the arteries. This belief is also false. Atherosclerosis is caused by inflammation. I will address the best ways to avoid inflammation later on in this book.

Cholesterol is a major building of life, without it the body cannot function optimally. The lie concerning cholesterol was created because pharmaceutical companies developed a way to " lower" it with the use of drugs. They then instructed all of their "pushers", the MD"s to prescribe this dangerous drug and facilitate this horrendous lie to the population of the world. Well I am not allowing that. I am telling the truth so that we can all live long and healthy lives.

In closing I'll ask you to consider two points. Point one, statins were introduced on the market in the early 1980's. By the end of the 1980's we see a spike in alzheimer's, which prior to, was a pretty obscure disease. Point 2, we as a people have been consuming animal flesh for more than 8000 thousand years. If it were bad for us, would not we have known before now. Edward Louis Bernays, the nephew of Sigmund Freud and "father of propaganda" once said " I do not have to convince the american people of anything, I simply must convince their MD"s. The people will follow." He made that statement in response to a campaign in the late 1920's that he created to get american women hooked on cigarettes. Let that sink in.

The Truth About Supplements

According to data collected by the Council for Responsible Nutrition, Americans spent 21 billions dollars on dietary supplements in 2015. The data showed that upwards of 68% of Americans took some type of dietary supplement, with 84% expressing confidence in the product that they were consuming. The age group with the highest percentage of supplement users was 18-34 (66%) with this group anticipating that their overall supplement use would likely increase over the next five years. Most supplement users, 87% do their best to eat a well balanced diet, 76% have regular doctor visits and 67% believe that exercise is a critical part of health. On paper these numbers seem excellent Americans not only seem to be conscious of their health but also willing to take a responsible role in maintaining that health, however a closer look reveals some startling details.

As of 2015 an estimated 160 million Americans were considered obese, with 30% being under the age of 20. A 2015 study revealed that 55% of Americans are taking pharmaceutical drugs. Between 1997 and 2016 the number of prescriptions filled for both children and adults rose from 2.4 billion to 4.5 billion. An article published in Newsweek in 2014 took a look at a different study that compared the overall health of 11 countries, including the US, France, Canada, and Norway, just to name a few. Researchers found that the US ranked last in all areas pertaining to health. How is this possible; how is it that Americans are spending so much much and effort into being healthy, but clearly the overall health of the country is declining? Well, let's take a look at two more studies. The first study, published in 2018, took place between 2007 and 2016. The study found that many over the counter supplements contained ingredients in prescription medications, anabolic steroids and banned pharmaceutical drugs. The study looked at 800 different supplements. Finally, a study published in 2013 found that 33% of supplements tested did not contain the supplement that was advertised and another 33% contained either less than the proclaimed amount of the supplement or the supplement was in an inorganic, man made form that the human body simply could not use. Simply stated, Americans are now spending upwards of 35 billion dollars every year, for supplements that are not what they are advertised to be. Americans are being legally robbed.

There are many problems with supplements and supplement companies in America, so let's take a look at a few of the major problems. The first problem is that supplements are not regulated. A supplement company is free to make virtually any claim about their product and what it does, and their claims do not have to be true. As long as the packaging or commercial states "These statements have not been evaluated by the FDA" then they pretty much have free reign over what they can say. The second problem with most supplement companies is quality control. From the person who extracts the vitamin from the plant in South America, to the person who finally bottles the product is a extremely long process and most companies quality control is not efficient enough to ensure that what they claim is in the bottle, is actually in the bottle. A third major problem with these companies is the recipe. Let me explain it this way. I love my Grandmother's apple pie, it is for me, by far the best dessert ever, much better than anything store bought. Why is that? It is due to the freshness of the ingredients and the recipe. For instance, if a supplement company does not have just the right amount of calcium and just the right amount of Iron, then the Calcium will prevent the absorption of the Iron; or if either are in form that the body can not use then it also can not be absorbed. Let me give you an example. Calcium Carbonate is a form of calcium that the human body, for the most part, can not absorb. That's because Calcium Carbonate is basically chalk; but in my opinion the worst thing about supplement companies is that for the most part, all research done on their products have been conducted in house, meaning they paid for the research. You do not need to be a scientist to see that there exist a serious conflict of interest. All of these factors work to create an environment that facilitates a depreciation of health for the average American who believes that he or she is taking a useful product. If you can not pronounce the words on your supplement label, then those are probably drugs.

So, am I saying that all supplements are bad, or there is no need for supplements? Absolutely not, on the contrary. I believe that due to how food is produced in America, that everyone of us would be prudent to take some type of dietary supplement. The questions to ask are, what type of supplements are actually necessary and which ones do not contain pharmaceutical drugs or anabolic steroids. Let's look at a few types. The first is protein powders. For the most part , the average American, athlete or non athlete, does not need to supplement with protein powders. It is quite easy to get all the protein that the body requires with food only. Not to mention that not all protein powders are absorbable, and the biggest factor, why isn't this product molding? Yes molding, if a protein powder is made of whey (milk) or Egg, or plants, then why isn't it molding, because all those things mold. What chemical is in that product that is preventing it from molding? The second useless supplement is pre workouts. Pre Workouts are said to provide you with energy for your workout, but isn't that what food is supposed to do? If you lack energy then you lack B Vitamins, these are the Vitamins responsible for metabolising the food that you eat into energy, but also remember, gluten prevents the absorption of all nutrients, so you may want to eliminate gluten first, and then energy will not be a problem anymore. The final useless supplement that I will discuss are fat burners. Let me explain why. Let's first understand what fat is, and how and why does the body store it. There are only three foods on earth. Regardless of what sub categories may exist all foods are either protein, carbohydrates or fats. Basically, if it is any kind of animal it is a protein. If it grew from the earth it is a carbohydrate. Fats are different, they exist as proteins or carbs. They do not have their category. For instance salmon and tuna are both considered to be fats. While avocado and most nuts are fats also. When it comes to storage, the human body does not store fat. I will repeat that, the human body does not store fat. Remember, your brain, nervous system, sex hormones and every cell membrane in your body are made of fat, and you are in a constant state of regeneration every moment of your life. Your body uses and metabolizes fat at an high rate. Your body also does not store protein. Once your amino acid pool is full, the body simply discards of all excess protein. The only nutrient that the body stores is carbohydrates. Why? Because carbs are fuel to the body. Carbs and fats are made of the exact same molecules that are arranged differently.

When you eat an excessive amount of carbs, then the body simply rearranges the molecules into fat and stores it within pre existing fats cells. Your body is doing the same thing that you would if gasoline were free for the next 24 hours. You would fill every container that you could and store that gas aka food aka energy for a "rainy day." So excess body fat is nothing more than stored energy and physics teachers us that energy cannot be burned, it must be used. The only fat burner that works efficiently and safely with no possible health risks, is activity. You have to get up and actually do something.

So what types of supplements do I recommend? Good question. I recommend supplements that support the overall health, structure and function of the human body. Things like Vitamins, Omega 3,6,9 , Minerals, herbs, roots and any other truly natural substances. These are the substances that the body can absorb and easily use. These are the things that produce vitality.

In the midst of so many bad supplement companies there are a few really good ones that provide products that do what they claim to do and really help the human body. Time does not permit me to speak about all of them, however I will briefly speak on the two that I trust and personally use. The first company is Youngevity. Youngevity was founded by Dr Joel Wallach an N.D. with more than 50 years of experience. His products were developed from data he collected from 10,000 autopsies, and over 1 million blood chemistries and histopathologies that he performed. Simply stated, he put in a lot of work and research into the development of Youngevity. All of his research was funded by the USDA, which means its data can be trusted, especially since it contradicts what the USDA considers healthy today. His products range from Fish oil, supplements for bone and joint health, healthy brain packs, Selenium, a mineral associated with the prevention of cancer, and plant derived minerals. I have been using and recommending Youngevity for many years and I have only seen positive results. The second company that I highly recommend is called Life One. Life One is an herbal supplement that is marketed as an immune system booster. This is wonderful because the ultimate cause of any disease is ultimately a failure of the immune system. In America I cannot tell you that eliminating the 12 bad foods and supplementing with life one cures cancer. It is illegal for anyone to make such a claim, so I will not make any claim of that matter. I do however highly recommend this product to everyone regardless of your current health.

When it comes to supplements you must remember that at the other end of that bottle is a for profit company. A company that may or may not be ethical and care about your health. It is a simple application of "buyer beware." The last person to tell you how good a product is, is the person who made it. In some cases they have a invested reason to lie.

How To Read Food Labels

Understanding how to decipher the the information on food labels and packaging is vital to the individual who wants to take control of their health beginning with nutrition. We have all heard the old saying that you are what you eat, and we all know this to be true, but the question is, what are we eating? America has the highest GDP of any country on earth, that just means that we have a lot of money, yet we are 43 in the world as it pertains to life expectancy. We trail countries that we consider third world like South korea and Taiwan when it comes to how long we live. We go to MD's for health advice and their life expectancy is lower than the national average. The rates of cancer, alzheimer's, autism and just about every other chronic disease has risen since 1900. Clearly, we have missed something. What we have done is given away our power to food manufactures. We believe their labels, we believe their marketing, we believe that the product must be good or the

FDA would not allow it to be sold, we believe whatever they say with no regard.

When it comes to food manufactures we must adopt the same "buyer beware" mindset that we employ with supplement companies. This is wholly due to the FDA, they allow manufactures to lie, to put chemicals into our foods and there is no repercussions for it. In October 2018, after nearly 50 years of allowing certain chemicals into the US food supply the FDA finally banned - anibenzophenone (benzophenone) -ethyl acrylate, -eugenyl methyl ether (methyl eugenol), -myrcene, - pulegone and-pyridine. All of these poisons cause cancer and the FDA has known that for decades. The ironic things is that food manufactures have two full years to comply. The FDA is a joke organization that cares nothing about your health and the sooner that you realize that, the sooner you will take back your power and educate yourself on what you are eating.

So what I want to do is share with you a few tips and insight into reading food labels and a few things to look for on those labels and packaging. However, before I begin I want to give you my disclaimer. It is impossible for me to list every bad thing that is added to foods in America. First, it's just to much. Second the FDA does not allow food manufacturers to disclose chemicals that they add. They are only required to list "food Stuff" which is a FDA term for chemicals that they call food. So neither I, nor any other health care professional even knows whats all in manufactured foods. For that cause, I recommend that you simply do not shop at grocery stores, especially the large chain stores. Why do business with a company who knowing and willingly, for profit, sells you poison? In my home, we do not shop at grocery stores for anything other than things like salt, baking soda, gluten free flour and small things like that. Otherwise, we shop at local farms, farmers markets and local butchers.

When it comes to understanding food labels you must begin with an understanding that the label is in two parts. The front side and the back side aka the marketing side and the government side. On the marketing side you may see words such as "Healthy" "Smart" "Gluten Free" " Natural" "Zero" "Low" etc etc. These words mean nothing. They are defined by what the FDA says that they are and not Webster's dictionary. For instance, it is impossible for anything food or drink on earth, except water, to have zero calories. Zero sugar means that the sweeteners are chemicals and not real sugar. I'm sure that everyone has seen the little white mushrooms that grow randomly in the grass. Those are all natural, and they are also all poison. Zero trans fat is an illusion because trans fat is not an ingredient that can be added. It is a by product of heating partially hydrogenated oil. Everything about the front of any food package is there to cause you to want to purchase that product. It's only marketing. You have never seen the world healthy on a bag of apples. That's because things that are healthy, natural or smart do not need to advertise.

The government side of the label is the side that the FDA regulates what the manufacturer must include, what information must be available to the consumer. We already know what that information is, it's the foods nutritional values and ingredients, which includes "food stuff." These include not only the list that I shared earlier, but also things like yellow and red #4, which are illegal in every country in the world except for the US, monosodium glutamate, which has a severe impact on cognitive functions but also chemicals like calcium silicate, which is used in powders as an anticaking agent and table salt, but also as a safe alternative to asbestos in high temperature insulation materials.

Let's briefly return to supplement labels as well. The government side of a supplement has its nutritional values as well. The label will say things like "Vitamin A in the form of beta carotene." Let me explain what this means. All vitamins have precursors. The precursors are found in foods. You eat the food and your body converts the precursor into the vitamin. So what that means is there is no vitamin A in that product. There is a man made , synthetic version of the precursor in the product, that your body may or may not absorb. Similarly, you may read "calcium in the form of calcium carbonate." Calcium is a mineral. Minerals come from the soil and transferred into plants. Either you eat the plant, or you eat the animal that ate the plant, and that's how you get minerals into your body. So, the statement about calcium means the exact same thing. It means that there is a man made, synthetic version of the mineral, that your body may or may not be able to absorb.

Understanding food labels can be a daunting task but it is a task that is necessary. The amount of poisons and toxins that are put into our foods is a major contributor to the decline of the health of people everywhere on earth and particularly here in the US. My answer to this dilemma is simple, don't support the large chain stores. Shop local farms and local butchers, and fisherman. Not only will it improve your health but it will help your local economy. Remember, you are what you eat, but if you can't even pronounce the words, then what are you really eating?

The Science of Breathing

As a human being you breathe about 23,000 times per day, nearly 8.5 million times per year. Yet, in the west, we take no thought about how our breath affects our overall physical health and mental state of being. We do this because we are not taught the importance of our breath nor how it literally affects our brains.. We are taught to listen to our MD, because the MD knows what's best for our health and wellbeing; but consider this, yogis, martial artist, law enforcement and military snipers are all taught how to breathe. Allow me to teach you how to breathe.

Using a functional brain scan we discover that the human brain is a electromagnetic machine that emits five distinct brain waves. These brain waves are gamma, which is a super conscious state, beta, which is your normal conscious state, alpha, which is a very relaxed, not thinking state. Theta, which is the "dream" or meditative state, and delta, which is the sleep state. Now, I want to keep this simple and not get into a ton of neuroscience, so just understand that the state that your brain is in controls every aspect of your life, and your breathe largely controls the state of your brain.

So here is what I want you to do. Take a deep breath. Inhale and exhale deeply. Did your shoulders move up on the inhale, kind of like you got a little taller and then come back down on the exhale? If so then you are what Dr. Belisa Vranich calls a vertical breather, and it is a really horrible way to breathe. Let me explain. When you breath in this way you are breathing from the smallest portion of your lungs, the top, but the most oxygen rich portion is in the lower parts of your lungs. The second issue that you are not using your diaphragm, the muscle that is designed to help you breathe. You are , however using your neck and shoulders, muscles that were never designed to be breathing muscles. So if you have neck pain of any kind, then improper breathing has played its role in that ailment. Next, because you are breathing from the part of your lungs with the least amount of oxygen, that means that in order to get enough oxygen in then you have to breath faster than you normally would. This type of breathing puts your brain in a high beta state, which is the equivalent to you encountered by a lion in the wild, that wants to eat you. Your breathe makes your brain believe that you are in a fight or flight situation. Once that happens your body releases adrenaline and cortisol. These are the stress hormones and your body releases them in preparation to run away. The human body is designed with this safety system in place, and it works well, but only when the stress response is acute and not chronic. Here's why, once in that state your physiology has to change. Blood is pushed from your internal organs into your arms and legs. Once this happens your body has ceased to be in growth and is now in protection. All systems of regeneration are shut down as the body prepares to mobilize. The next thing that happens is that blood is pushed from the prefrontal cortex, the place of rational thinking, into the midbrain, the primitive part of the brain associated with motor skills. So a flaw in breathing not only pushes you out of growth and into protection but it also literally lowers your intelligence: and all of that is ok, if the response lasts for a few minutes, after that the body can go back to its normal physiological state and everything continues on. However, if this state is chronic, meaning it persists on and on and on without any ending, then your body is literally in a state of perpetual death. All because of a perceived threat due to improper breathing.

So how did this happen? How is it even possible to do something as natural as breathing so wrong? Well, I think that it was and is done by design. Look at a child under the age of 5 years old or an animal. They breath horizontally not vertically. They both are using their diaphragm to breathe, so improper breathing is something that you learned, so it is something that you can unlearn.

In the west children start school at 5 years old. They spend up to 10 hours a day in a classroom seated at a desk, and this continues at least for the next 12 years, assuming that the child completes high school. Well it's this sitting all day that encourages bad posture. Sitting for extended periods of time causes you to lean forward and slouch. For this position you collapse the rib cages and lungs into a position that makes breathing horizontally extremely difficult, so by default, because we still need to breathe, we begin to breathe vertically, from our chest, and over time this abnormal breathing becomes easier and easier because we repeat the pattern so often. So by the time we are in our 20's and 30's ,we've forgotten what it feels like to breathe correctly and even more damaging, we have now been running from the lion everyday since we were about 7 years old.

Here is a quick exercise to teach you how to breathe. Perform this exercise 10 minutes every day for as long as it takes to recreate your breathing pattern. From a standing position, maintaining good posture, violently breathe out your mouth, while sucking in your stomach, then violently breathe in expanding your stomach. This will retrain your body to use your diaphragm to breathe and to quit relying on your chest. Once you have mastered breathing, you can truly begin to heal your mind and body as you will have freed yourself from the agitated brain state of constant beta waves.

"So now let's consider, what is a mind in the grip of vicious circles.......................... One of the most obvious instances that we all know is the phenomenon of worry.......... The Doctor tells you that you have to have an operation, and that has been set up so that automatically everyone worries about it,..... but since worry takes away your appetite and your sleep, it's not good for you. But you can't stop worrying and therefore you get additionally worried that you are worried...................., and then furthermore, because that is quite absurd and you are mad at yourself because you do it,.................... you are worried because you worry because you worry; and that is a vicious circle................ So can you allow your mind to be quiet?........ Isn't it difficult, because the mind seems to be like a monkey....jumping up and down and jabbering all of the time. Once you have learned to think, you just can't stop."   Alan Watts

In the movie The Matrix, Neo, the main character, is given two options. Take one pill and life goes on as it always has. Take a different colored pill and you wake up and see how things really are, and what the truth really is. While I am sure that there are many who believe that this movie is science fiction, I'm here to tell you that it is not.....it's a documentary.

Quantum Physics, Neuroscience and Epigenetics all point to several overwhelming truths about all of mankind. The first truth is that we have all been programmed. The second truth is that, regardless of what we want and desire on a conscious level, that it is the subconscious programs that are controlling our lives, and the third truth is that we all have the power within ourselves to change the programs at anytime and thus change our lives. Now I know that some of you may say that you are not programmed, you may say that you are in complete and conscious control, and you may be. You may have come to the truth of the knowledge that I am about to present, however, for the vast majority, most of this will be foreign.

Within the first seven years of life, and in particular, the first four, we are all programmed. We come into this world with no preconceived ideas or thoughts about anything. Everything that we come to know, we know because someone taught it to us. How else do you believe that you learned to talk? The people closest to us, in most cases our parents, were the ones that installed the programs. These are the basic building blocks for how we think, and we know that how we think controls what we experience from life. The powers that be understand this concept exceptionally well. Why do you think that whenever some horrific event happens they play it on every news channel, every day, all day , for weeks and weeks? They are programming you to be fearful, a fear, extreme beta, state of mind renders you powerless. That's how they control you, through programming. The Jesuits knew this 400 years ago. That's why they said, "Give me us a child until he is seven years old , and he will belong to the church forever."

Consider this, 95% of your day, your life is being controlled by your subconscious mind, and your subconscious mind is controlled by the programs. Which are controlled by your conscious mind, this is the mind that runs the day to day activity, the mind that says, "Hey, I want this out of life." That mind is only in control of 5% of your day. So the interesting fact is this, until you change your subconscious programs then you can never change your life because when the subconscious and conscious mind do not agree with one another, then the subconscious mind always wins. We know this because Psychologist have shown that 90% of the programs that have been passed down to us, do not serve our best interest. Ok, so how do we reprogram the subconscious mind? One way that I am sure that everyone has heard of is affirmations. The repetitiveness of anything will create a change in the subconscious mind. If you are however making these affirmations while in a beta state of mind then you are doing things the hard way. Allow me to digress for a moment. The reason that the first seven years of life is when the programs are installed most effectively, is because in the first seven years of life, your mind is in a constant theta state. You are in a state of hypnosis and plugged directly into your subconscious mind. The programs do not pass through any interference. Again, this is how the powers that be program you with the news. The waves from the television take your mind into a theta state, where you are prepped and ready to be programmed with whatever delusion that they want you to believe.

The key to life is then, to identify the programs that no longer serve who you are and who you want to be, and then install new programs that allow you to attract everything that you want to experience from life. So, now how do you do that? You do so by entering a theta state of mind. Remember, theta is a state of self hypnosis, it's the "dream state." In theta you will be able to tap into your memories and uninstall those unwanted programs, and then using your affirmations you can install your new affirmations. Simply put, you go into meditation. The benefits of meditation are very well documented so i will not go into a lot of science about this. That information is easily accessible to anyone. I will however list some of the known benefits.

Reduced Stress

Better Control over Anxiety

Emotional Health

Self Awareness

Better Attention Span

Reduced Age Related Memory Loss

Breaks Addictions

Improved Sleep

Lower Blood Pressure

These are not the only benefits, there are many more. Instead of trying to explain how to meditate and get into a theta state, I will leave some resources and video links in the "Helpful Resources" section at the end of this book. I am going to leave you with three techniques that bring synchronicity to both hemispheres of the brain, doing this takes you into an alpha state of mind which is also very powerful and a good state to speak your affirmations into, there is less resistance from the conscious mind in alpha as well.

The first technique is known as brain gym. Brain gym is simply understanding that the left hemisphere of the brain controls the right side of the body and the right hemisphere controls the left side. So what you do is simply cross your arms and or legs. By doing this you engage both hemispheres at the same time creating hemi sync. The last two techniques are breathing techniques. They are breathing rhythm patterns. The first is a 4-8-8-4 breathing pattern, and the second is a 3-6-6-3 pattern. Both patterns work this way. Breathe in for 4 seconds, hold for 8, exhale for 8 seconds and then hold for 4 seconds. The same pattern applies to 3-6-6-3. All three techniques create hemi sync in the brain, which as I stated earlier, will get you into an alpha brain state.

"So in the same way that a muddy, turbulent pool quiets itself when left alone, you have to know how to leave your mind alone…….it will quiet itself."

Alan Watts

WHAT IS

EARTHING

According to recent research from both Harvard and Yale schools of medicine, inflammation is the root cause of all chronic disease. I am sure that we have all heard the term inflammation, but what is it. Well, if we break you down into tiny pieces, you will find that you are made up of protons, which have a positive charge, neutrons, which have a neutral charge, and electrons which have a negative charge.Inflammation occurs when an atom loses an electron. That atom is then said to be a free radical, and free radicals cause oxidative damage. Let me give you a practical example. Iron beginning to rust is an example of oxidative damage. Look back to the Chapter on Cholesterol, at the end of page 12. I began to speak on this oxidative damage at that time. Ok, so let's briefly recap. Inflammation is the cause of all chronic disease, and inflammation happens when a atom loses an electron and becomes a free radical. On earth we live inside of a battery. Protons and electrons are deposited into our onosphere. (the surface 40 to 50 miles above the earth) The protons remain above the earth, giving the ionosphere a positive charge and electrons are deposited into the earth via lightning strikes, giving the earth a negative charge. We live inside of a battery.

Earthing is simply placing your bare feet upon the earth. In doing so you absorb electrons into the body through the soles of your feet. This is a very ancient practice. The Native Americans would have the children wet their moccasins before dancing around the fire. This is because leather, when wet, is a great conductor of electricity. If we look at the indigenous people all over the earth, the people who still walk predominately barefoot, you do not see all of the sickness and disease that you see in the west. Their bodies are not inflamed to the point of oxidative damage.

While earthing is an ancient practice, there is also science based research that has been done that proves the claims made by proponents of earthing. The work began with Drs Karol and Pawel Sokal in Poland and continued with Clint Ober in the US. Since then there have been twenty five studies and ten commentaries written on the health benefits of earthing. Dr. Jeff Spencer credits earthing will all the success that he and his athletes experienced during not one Tour De France victory, but eight. There are many benefits of earthing including, but not limited to

Stress Relief

Sports performance

Healing Properties

Reduced Pain

Speeds healing

Lowers Inflammation

the list is literally limitless. For anyone interested in reading any of the studies or commentaries, I will leave a link in the Helpful Resources section at the end of the book.

I understand that asking someone to go and stand in the grass for 6 to 8 hours a day may not be achievable for everyone. Maybe you do not have the time to do it, or maybe you live in a city where you just are not going to find much grass to stand in. What do you do? Well, the Earthing Institute sells earthing products from sheets, that you sleep on. Floor matts for those of you who have desk jobs, and a wide variety of other earthing tools. I use a earthing sheet and I can tell you that it was one of the best investments that I have ever made. I will also leave links to where you can purchase these products in the Helpful Resources section.

You Are Water

In 1994 Dr. Masaru Emoto performed his famous water experiment. Dr Emoto would take water from the tap, rivers and lakes. He would then place the water from one source into multiple jars. On each jar , he would write a word like, Love, or hate. Peace or war. He would also play music played in 432 hz for one jar of water and music played in 440 hz for a different jar. He would pray healing prayers to one jar and prayers of hate to another jar. He would only do one thing at a time to any jar of water. For instance, there may be four jars of the same tap water, and four jars of river water, etc, etc. He would test the tap water separately from the river water. The way that the experiment would go is he would go is that he would have his four test jars and one control jar. The control would not be exposed to anything. He would expose the water to these various environments over night, and then he would freeze the water and observe the crystals under a microscope. What he found was that the water exposed to loving words, kind prayers and music in 432 hz produced beautiful crystals, distinct from the control jar. He found that water exposed to hateful words, hateful prayers, and music in 440 hz produced very undesirable crystals. What this means is that intention has a powerful effect on water. Why should you care; because your body is 70% water.

Water is the most abundant natural resource that we have on earth. Water covers 70% of the earth's surface area, and quite frankly, it is impossible for life to exist in the absence of water. The powers that be would have you believe that there is a lack of water, this is false, there is no lack of water or anything for that matter. Every place on earth where there is a mountain range, the earth is producing fresh water every single day. So particularly here in the US, lack of water is not an issue. The issue is clean water.

The United States of America is the last country one might consider when speaking of the availability of clean drinking water, however that is a problem that almost every American faces.

A study conducted from 1982 to 2015 found that nearly 45 million Americans, annually are exposed to were exposed to unsafe drinking water. The study, conducted by Maura Allaire, an urban planner at the University of California-Irvine, found that fecal coliform, inorganic arsenic, inorganic lead, inorganic fluoride, pharmaceutical drugs, and several other inorganic chemicals were present in the water. Inorganic simply means that all of these were were man made, not natural. This is serious, and if unchecked will create help create chronic health problems in a large portion of our population. So what do we do ? Before you think anything political, please understand that no politician is going to help you. If they were then they would have done so already. This is your responsibility and you have to do something about it for yourself.

I have purchased a used several water filters. In the Helpful Resources, I will put links to these two that I think worked the best. The water that you drink is important ……..remember, you are water.

CONCLUSION

First, allow me to take the opportunity to personally thank you for not only purchasing my EBook "VITALITY" but also for reading it. I wrote this Ebook to help you live a holistically healthy life and I few a more resources that i would like to share. So below you will find links to free information on meditation. You will find the video that I used to learn how to reach a theta state. You will find links to several books that I have read that have helped me greatly, and you will links to all of the products that I mentioned. I personally use all of the products below and I highly recommend that you do as well. They have helped me and my family gain Vitality and I pray that they help you as well……..

Namaste.

HELPFUL RESOURCES

MEDITATION LINKS

The Mindful Awareness Research Center at UCLA provides a set of meditations on its website.

The Wild Divine channel on YouTube offers lots of short guided meditations, from the likes of Deepak Chopra, Andrew Weil, Dean Ornish, and Nawang Khechog.

Learning Meditation Meditation Room has a whole variety of meditations available. Some of them sound a bit corporate to me, but I like most of them. I love the voice of the guy who does "Fulfill Your Own Potential"—he sounds to me like some grizzled old woodland spirit

LINK TO YOUTUBE MEDITATION VIDEO

https://www.youtube.com/watch?v=Xr5dkZhLtRM HYPERLINK "https://www.youtube.com/watch?v=Xr5dkZhLtRM&list=PLD8L-goGbAOcx1Doirw-Z2u5m_waq5xuk" HYPERLINK "https://www.youtube.com/watch?v=Xr5dkZhLtRM HYPERLINK "https://www.youtube.com/watch?v=Xr5dkZhLtRM&list=PLD8L-goGbAOcx1Doirw-Z2u5m_waq5xuk"& HYPERLINK "https://www.youtube.com/watch?v=Xr5dkZhLtRM&list=PLD8L-goGbAOcx1Doirw-Z2u5m_waq5xuk"list=PLD8L-goGbAOcx1Doirw-Z2u5m_waq5xuk" HYPERLINK "https://www.youtube.com/watch?v=Xr5dkZhLtRM&list=PLD8L-goGbAOcx1Doirw-Z2u5m_waq5xuk"& HYPERLINK "https://www.youtube.com/watch?v=Xr5dkZhLtRM&list=PLD8L-goGbAOcx1Doirw-Z2u5m_waq5xuk" HYPERLINK "https://www.youtube.com/watch?v=Xr5dkZhLtRM HYPERLINK "https://www.youtube.com/watch?v=Xr5dkZhLtRM&list=PLD8L-goGbAOcx1Doirw-Z2u5m_waq5xuk"& HYPERLINK "https://www.youtube.com/watch?v=Xr5dkZhLtRM&list=PLD8L-goGbAOcx1Doirw-Z2u5m_waq5xuk"list=PLD8L-goGbAOcx1Doirw-Z2u5m_waq5xuk" HYPERLINK "https://www.youtube.com/watch?v=Xr5dkZhLtRM&list=PLD8L-goGbAOcx1Doirw-Z2u5m_waq5xuk"list=PLD8L-goGbAOcx1Doirw-Z2u5m_waq5xuk

LINK TO MY YOUTUBE VIDEO ON BREATHING RHYTHM PATTERNS

https://www.youtube.com/watch?v=8kgqYIyhkR4 HYPERLINK "https://www.youtube.com/watch?v=8kgqYIyhkR4&t=218s" HYPERLINK "https://www.youtube.com/watch?v=8kgqYIyhkR4 HYPERLINK "https://www.youtube.com/watch?v=8kgqYIyhkR4&t=218s"& HYPERLINK "https://www.youtube.com/watch?v=8kgqYIyhkR4&t=218s"t=218s" HYPERLINK "https://www.youtube.com/watch?v=8kgqYIyhkR4&t=218s"& HYPERLINK "https://www.youtube.com/watch?v=8kgqYIyhkR4&t=218s" HYPERLINK "https://www.youtube.com/watch?v=8kgqYIyhkR4 HYPERLINK "https://www.youtube.com/watch?v=8kgqYIyhkR4&t=218s"& HYPERLINK "https://www.youtube.com/watch?v=8kgqYIyhkR4&t=218s"t=218s" HYPERLINK "https://www.youtube.com/watch?v=8kgqYIyhkR4&t=218s"t=218s

LINK TO EARTHING RESEARCH

http://www.earthinginstitute.net/research/

LINK TO LIFEONE IMMUNITY SUPPLEMENT AND THE RESEARCH BEHIND IT, YOU CAN ALSO PURCHASE FROM THIS LINK

http://www.lifeone.org/

Here are several brands of gluten free flours that I use

https://amzn.to/2SgtBVp

https://amzn.to/2SheQl9

https://amzn.to/2P8mIn0

https://amzn.to/2TTCDJB

https://amzn.to/2TTdWx0

https://amzn.to/2P7se9y

Here are links to supplements that I personally use. The company is name Youngevity, and it was started by Dr Joel Wallach ND

This is a mineral supplement. It contains 60 essential minerals. The recommendation is one bottle per 100 pounds of bodyweight per month

https://amzn.to/2SjUOGR

This is glucogel. It is for bone and joint health. It contains glucosamine, so it is not recommended if you are allergic to shellfish. There are two different sizes

https://amzn.to/2TUKmqM

https://amzn.to/2P7sk0U

These are essential fatty acids. Omega 3,6,9

https://amzn.to/2E6CHkC

https://amzn.to/2P56mvH

These are multivitamins. They are for men and women and all ages.

https://amzn.to/2TV6amn

https://amzn.to/2Sj1xAW

This is selenium a trace mineral. Studies have shown that supplementing with selenium reduces the risk of some cancers by up to 80%

https://amzn.to/2Rrij0M

https://amzn.to/2P7MXKg

https://amzn.to/2KEZ54Y

This is a PUR advanced water filter. It is not the best but it it useful an affordable.

https://amzn.to/2Sj4IIC

This is a reverse osmosis water filter. This strips the water of all toxins.

https://amzn.to/2TV9jCr

This is a home master water filter. This one filters all of the water that comes into your home. Ideally, this is the best one.

https://amzn.to/2SjVpbz

This is a book by Dr Peter Glidden. It is titled

'The MD Emperor Has No Clothes: Everybody Is Sick and I Know Why"

Dr Glidden is an ND, in this book he explains why conventional medical practices are outdated and simply do not work.

https://amzn.to/2P7iCfa

'Dead Doctors Don't Lie

This book was written by Dr Joel Wallach ND. In this book Dr Wallach explains how to prevent and even cure over 400 diseases with the use of vitamins and minerals.

https://amzn.to/2RnxeJa

These are various earthing sheets and matts.

https://amzn.to/2ra2waU

https://amzn.to/2TTfQh8

https://amzn.to/2TTRp35

https://amzn.to/2ScZePy

https://amzn.to/2rbno1t

https://amzn.to/2KIfXb5

https://amzn.to/2KJXfA0

https://amzn.to/2TY9f5d

Shop Vitality Merchandise

https://teespring.com/stores/coach-mike-fitness

COPYRIGHT

VITALITY: A Holistic and Natural Approach to Health by Michael Jones

Published Michael Jones Charlotte NC 28213

ABOUT THE AUTHOR

Michael Jones started his sports and athletic career at the age of six years old. Since then he has been an Elite three sport athlete, participating in Football, Baseball and Boxing at the highest amateur levels, while also being invited to attend the 2005 NFL Football Scouting Combine. Michael has two degrees. One in Nutrition and the other Sports Management and Exercise Science and also holds four globally recognized fitness certifications. With over ten years of training experience he has trained over 300 High

School, Collegiate and Professional athletes from various sports. Michael has also trained more than 10000 non athlete clients, ranging from the 18 year old high school student to the 81 year old grandmother. Michaels training philosophy centers around improving functional movement of the human body and thus increasing a person's performance, whether that performance is in the world of athletics or everyday life. Michael has also studied Complementary and Alternative medicine and believes that all disease arise as a result of dysfunction in one of the body systems and these dysfunctions can be remedied, in all cases, without the use of pharmaceutical drugs. Michaels dedication to correcting the human movement system, while also improving cardiovascular function and building lean muscle has led him to adopt the ideology that " if you move better, then you feel better and if you feel better then you live better

Made in the USA
Columbia, SC
02 December 2018